When Push Comes To Shove's Guide To Social Services

Your Rights & How To Navigate The System

NICKITA STARCK

ISBN: 9798838498182

This book provides general information for interest only and does not replace official advice. Whilst every effort has been made to ensure the content is accurate, the author accepts no liability or responsibility for any loss or damage caused or thought to be caused, by making choices based upon the contents of this book and recommends that you use it in conjunction with other trusted sources.

Cover design - Nickita Starck / Image - Canva

DEDICATION

This book is dedicated to my dear friend and mentor Beverley Beech. Without her love, support and belief in me, my life would be very different.

CONTENTS

ACKNOWLEDGMENTS

I have so many people to thank who have helped me along my journey. My dear husband Matt has supported me through thick and thin against all odds. He has held space for me to be me and ultimately help so many women.

I want to thank my dear team of telegram admins who have worked so hard to grow When Push Comes To Shove. Rachel, Charlotte, Nikki, Jo, Alex, Sheryl, Mike, Morwenna and Maria. I want to thank you from the bottom of my heart for your love and support.

I also want to say a special thank you for Dr Tess Lawrie from the World Council for Health. Your belief in my message to women has given me the strength to speak up and continue my mission with integrity and confidence.

Finally I want to acknowledge my two daughters, Sophie & Dottie. If it were not for you wonderful souls, I would never have taken this path. You have taught me more than I ever dreamed was possible. You are my earth angels and I feel blessed that you chose me.

“Peace on earth begins at birth” Jeannine Parvati Baker

1 INTRODUCTION

My name is Nickita Starck and I am the founder of 'When Push Comes To Shove'. I founded this company, because to put it quite simply, it was critical! After years of fighting a broken maternity system, I decided the system works perfectly well for the system, just not the women birthing inside it. So I created a new one. When Push Comes To Shove is an alternative, natural, maternity structure.

I am inundated with emails asking for help because an unjustified referral has been made to Social Services. This is why I have written this short book. It can be severely traumatising to deal with Social Services, especially during such a vulnerable time in your life.
I hope this book will help provide clarity, assist you to navigate the system and ultimately empower you. If you need further support, please don't hesitate to contact me:
info@whenpushcomestoshove.co.uk

2 WHY ARE REFERRALS MADE?

First of all we must understand why a referral has occurred.

Anyone can make a referral if they are concerned with the wellbeing of your child. Hospitals and birth centres for example will have strict procedures for Child Protection Policy. Some women find themselves in a position where an individual healthcare worker has made a referral to Social Services as they have 'concerns' for the wellbeing of their baby. These concerns are determined by perception or, in many cases, mis-perception.

We live in a society which dictates the acceptable social 'norms'. If you do not fit into this category you may be flagged as a safeguarding risk. There are, of course, genuine reasons for Social Services referrals, domestic abuse for example (although 'genuine' is a matter of perception which can become quite convoluted). I am here to give you a comprehensive guide to how the system works and what you can do should you come up against an 'unjustified' referral.

I am not here to define what justified is, just to guide you in the right direction to help you navigate a very complicated and often subjective system.

There will always be people who choose to live 'differently' and they are often vilified for their life choices. The pandemic has been a catalyst of change for many people. People are asking more questions about whether or not the 'system' has our best interests at heart, and many have come to the conclusion that they no longer wish to engage in such a system. More and more women are choosing to freebirth (unassisted childbirth), due to a previous traumatic birth experience which they feel was a result of systemic practice in the first place. Wanting to avoid such trauma, by eliminating the cause of the first unnecessary agonising experience, for many, will seem like common sense. However, it is often perceived differently by Health Professionals. They may view it as an 'extreme' option and may label such women as irresponsible. This is where phrases like 'what if something goes wrong?' are peppered into the conversation. This can be perceived as very coercive by some. They can feel disempowered and feel their innate ability to give birth is overlooked, and replaced by fear based, systemic, practice which does not take into consideration their previous trauma, or allow them to feel supported. Many women would like to engage mainstream care, but the fear of history repeating itself far outweighs the benefits of 'support', when they have a deep rooted belief that their body is perfectly capable of performing a physiological process without medical intervention. They are concerned that voicing their beliefs will in fact land them in deep water, so avoid the system altogether. The pandemic seems to have removed an open dialogue when it comes to making the right medical choices. As a result, some people can be coerced and bullied into a narrative where if they asked questions they would be shut down immediately.

I have received more emails and calls than I can count asking me for help due to Social Services referral for freebirthing. Many women feel that avoiding the system altogether is best for them, but situations do arise where they find themselves in the system unexpectedly. For example, if a woman was in labour and planning to freebirth but came across an issue/complication, she may wish to transfer to the hospital for help. This is arguably a sensible decision whereby the birthing woman has decided to engage help, for whatever reason, and health providers should note that as a caring and responsible action. This however is a romanticised notion and, even though a woman has changed her birth plans, due to unforeseen circumstances, she may still be flagged, possibly for 'concealing a pregnancy' or never having engaged with a Healthcare Provider.

Another example whereby a woman may be flagged is her lifestyle choices. For example, van life is becoming very popular in the UK. Many have chosen to leave the rat race and live a free and simple life either in a converted van or a boat. This will almost certainly raise a few eyebrows in the system as it is not deemed to be 'normal'.

They may think your child is at risk if you don't have running water for example. Boxes need to be ticked for them to be satisfied that your child has a safe environment to live in.

Another example would be that parents could be flagged for not being 'consumerists', meaning that they do not engage in a consumer lifestyle, and buy what they deem to be unnecessary products such as changing tables, cots and lots of baby products. Some may wish to co-sleep, change their baby's nappy on a simple towel, and lead a life outside the accepted narrative. Unfortunately, this can draw the attention of the authorities if they see this is a 'risk' to the baby. It can be viewed as 'weird' and non-compliant so will therefore put a target over the family.

As much as I wish I could offer you clear and concise law which will categorise what an 'at risk' child looks like, what their environment cannot look like and clear procedures thereafter, I cannot. This is a very grey area and referrals are at the mercy of the individual's perception of your life.

It will come down to what they perceive as normal and their interpretation of 'concern'. Even the process of referral can differ between trusts, and then how they are dealt with by local authorities, so all I can do is outline a typical policy and what you can do should you find yourself in this situation. The very fact that there is no clear legislation in place to determine how you can and cannot live can be a double- edged sword. On one hand the ambiguity works in your favour as they cannot quote any law that says for example 'you cannot free birth' but on the other hand, you cannot present them with a law that explains 'my lifestyle choices do not put my child at risk'.

There are laws that can give weight to your choices and protect you, but there is no clear cut answer.
I will do my best to provide clear and concise information so you are able to understand how the system works and what you can do to protect your family. I am not a lawyer so I cannot provide legal advice, I can only give you information so you can make an informed decision.

Before I get to policy, I want to draw upon my own experience over the years and offer some words of wisdom when it comes to how you actually conduct yourself with the authorities. This is crucial to understand so you do not inadvertently dig yourself a deeper hole. So I will make this 'point one' in my Guide to Navigating Social Services.

3 HOW TO CONDUCT YOURSELF

This is VERY important.
How you interact with Social Services can mean the difference between them cooperating with you or you just adding more fuel to the fire.
I have found that being contrary for the sake of it will only antagonise them. It is wonderful to have strong beliefs but you must understand that voicing what they perceive to be very 'alien' opinions will not help you. You must take a different approach. Just arguing your point and voicing your 'controversial' beliefs will not get them to understand. They have just as much chance of getting you to come round to their way of thinking in a short space of time. I am sure you will agree, that just is not going to happen!
First of all, take a deep breath, stay in trust and deal with this with a level head. Never make a decision from a place of fear, only love. Try to empathise with them. They are doing a job and inside every intimidating adult is a scared child. They are only people!

You must approach this with a cool head and love in your heart. They are not out to get you, they may have a genuine and personal concern due to their lenses of mis-perception. Accept that for what it is and focus on your approach. When you have a clear idea on how to conduct yourself, you will be able to deal with things on a step-by-step process and it will not seem so daunting

4 AVOIDING THEM IN THE FIRST PLACE

As the saying goes, the best form of self-defence is not to be in the fight in the first place.
So how do you avoid being on their radar? Many women contact me in early pregnancy expressing their wish to be out of the system completely. This is perfectly legal and you have every right to do so. Statistically if you are freebirthing for the right reasons, and NOT out of fear, the chances are you will have an amazing birth and there will be no need to enter the system. However, if you do need to engage their care for whatever reason, you may find yourself answering Social Services' questions. Ultimately, it is down to you to make an informed decision about how you navigate your care. If you feel the risk outweighs the benefit, then you are well within your rights to birth outside the system. Some women choose to 'have a toe' in the system to avoid any potential confrontation later down the line. They may want to attend antenatal visits, have scans

and blood tests if they choose to and decline intervention they do not consent to, then when it comes to the birth they may or may not decide to call the hospital for assistance.
Some choose to call the hospital after the baby has been born and they have established feeding. From a hospital perspective this is called a BBA (born before arrival). Some women find that this can work for them in the long run.

5 CHOOSE YOUR WORDING CAREFULLY

As I previously mentioned in point one, how you conduct yourself is everything. I will now share two examples of how you might want to 'word' your objections. Let us say for example, your baby has been born and you have received a letter with an appointment to have your baby vaccinated, but you do not wish for your baby to have these jabs after making an informed decision. There is no legal obligation to have your child vaccinated, but as I have already discussed, this could be perceived as a red flag, if you are already on their radar for freebirthing. For example: The trick is, not to be aggressive and not to voice all you know about potential adverse effects to vaccines. Consider asking them questions rather than explaining yourself and coming across as hostile and 'controversial'. Here is a template letter to decline such interventions.

Template letter - Step 1

Dear XXXX

Thank you for arranging a vaccination for XXX I do not have enough information to make an informed decision about this. I have a few questions before giving my consent.

1) For the above vaccination, what is the prevalence of the disease?
2) What is the mortality rate if the disease is contracted?
3) Is a doctor willing to sign an agreement that if XXX were vaccinated there would be no adverse/ severe reactions such as seizures, encephalopathy, persistent crying or severe fever?
4)May I please see the manufacturer's package insert 5) What are the chances of vaccine reaction over getting the actual disease itself? For example, it appears from some research a child is 6 times more likely to have a reaction to the DIP vaccination than the disease itself.
6) Why is a hep b vaccination being offered to a 2 month old? Hep b is contracted via semen, blood contaminated needles etc and the vaccination is only effective for about 10 years? I do not have hep b so she

could not contract it during birth. Why would a child need protection from an STD?
7) What percentage of adverse events are estimated to be reported to the yellow card scheme?
8.) If my child were to get these vaccinations, could she/he still get the disease that the vaccine is meant to protect?

I would be very grateful if my questions could be answered before the appointment time.

Kind regards

Template letter - step 2 (if you have received a response this letter may or may not be appropriate)

Dear XXX
I just wanted to put in writing confirmation that I do not consent to these vaccinations as I have thoroughly researched my options and made an informed decision.

The main reasons are as follows;

1) We have a vaccine related death in the family
(This may be relevant to you)

2) The emulsifiers used in the vaccines are polysorbate 80 which is linked to blood clots, strokes, heart attack and certain cancers. This emulsifier also allows the blood brain barrier to break, allowing any bacteria or viruses to enter the brain.

3) There is aluminium in the vaccine. A limit of 15-60μg has been derived by adjusting the adult imit to reflect the bodyweight of an infant. The UK schedule delivers 1,925μg to babies at 8 weeks, a further 800μg at 12 weeks, 1925μg at 16 weeks and more at 1 year. This is a worrying amount and it concerns me that this is not disclosed. Aluminium takes on a very different structure when injected. This is important for parents to know to make an informed decision.

4) Formaldehyde is an ingredient which can cause cancer

5) Sadly in response to my first letter, the doctor I spoke with did not have any answers to my questions. I am shocked that someone who actively encourages vaccinations would do so without any knowledge of ingredients and the interactions within a vaccine.
(This may or may not apply)

I would however like to thank the doctor for respecting my wishes and being so respectful and understanding of my decision as a parent. I trust I will not receive any more letters/reminders for this vaccination.

Kind regards

The following template letter could be used / adapted if you are a 'late booker'.

To [CONSULTANT MIDWIFE]

I just wanted to send you a courtesy email and introduce myself.
I am [?] weeks pregnant and very excited to meet my baby in [MONTH BABY IS DUE]. I have made an informed decision to self -refer to your maternity team. I am aware this is seen as 'late booking'. I have made the responsible decision to engage the optional service of NHS maternity care as I have suffered with a few ailments during my pregnancy and feel that the sensible thing to do is to engage extra support. I had previously engaged in private care but now feel I would like the support of the NHS.

I trust that when I meet your team I will be treated with compassion, kindness and understanding in line with the NHS Constitution, specifically;

"You have the right to receive care and treatment that is appropriate to you, meets your needs and reflects your preferences."

"You have the right not to be unlawfully discriminated against in the provision of NHS services including on grounds of gender, race, disability, age, sexual orientation, religion, belief, gender reassignment, pregnancy and maternity or marital or civil partnership status."

"You have the right to accept or refuse treatment that is offered to you, and not to be given any physical examination or treatment unless you have given valid consent."

I very much look forward to meeting your team and the support offered to me.

Kind regards

6 WHAT IS THE DEFINITION OF SAFEGUARDING?

The following is taken from cpdonline.co.uk *The definition of safeguarding, as per the Working Together to Safeguard Children Legislation, is:*

- Protecting children from maltreatment
- Preventing impairment of children's health or development.
- Ensuring that children are growing up in circumstances consistent with the provision of safe and effective care.
- Taking action to enable all children to have the best outcomes.

There are many different policies and legislation out there regarding safeguarding children, as it is such a fundamental aspect of education and childcare.

The key pieces of legislation that you might be aware of are:

- The Children Act 2004 (as amended).
- The Children and Social Work Act 2017.
- Keeping Children Safe in Education 2021

- Working Together to Safeguard Children 2018.
- The Education Act 2011.
- The United Nations convention on the Rights of the Child 1992.
- The Equality Act 2010.
- The Children and Families Act 2014.
- The Human Rights Act 1998.

7 FREE BIRTH & THE LAW

It is entirely legal for a woman to give birth without the attendance of a midwife or a doctor. You are not legally obligated to accept any medical care during pregnancy and birth nor can you be compelled to access care unless you lack the mental capacity to make decisions for yourself. (Birthrights 2017) You can find more information here:

RCM Clinical Briefing Sheet: 'freebirth' or 'unassisted childbirth' during the COVID-19 pandemic -

https://www.rcm.org.uk/media/3923 / freebirth_draft_30-april-v2.pdf

A midwife or healthcare professional should NOT be making Social Services referrals purely on the basis that a mother has declined medical care (Birthrights 2017) However, please understand it is illegal for anyone other than a qualified professional to assume the role of a midwife according to Article 45 of The Nursing And Midwifery Order (2001). To do so is a criminal offence. It is perfectly fine for other family members, friends or Doulas to be present at a freebirth, so long as they are not 'acting as a midwife'. It is not particularly clear in any legislation what 'Acting as a Midwife' entails. The following is a response from the NMC (Nursing And Midwifery Council) with their answer to this Question:

> Attendance of unqualified persons at childbirth
>
> *You have asked us to provide information about the Act and Regulation which provides further detail about attendance at childbirth.*
> *There is only one level of involvement as a midwife in childbirth itself, as this is a protected function under Article 45 of the Nursing and Midwifery Order 2001. This means that it is an offence for any person who is not a registered midwife or a registered medical practitioner to attend (please see definitions below) a woman in childbirth, except in an emergency or as part of approved training for those professions. We have produced information about Practising as a midwife (NMC 2017, updated 2021)*

The following excerpt from Practising as a Midwife provides further detail about the protected title and protected functions of midwives:

> *"Protected title and protected function*
> *Midwifery is regulated as a distinct profession. The title of 'midwife' is protected in law and there is a protected legal function associated with this title. It is an offence for someone to practise as a midwife while not registered, to falsely claim to have a midwifery qualification, or to use the title 'midwife' when not entitled to do so. Only those recorded on the NMC's register as holding a qualification in midwifery may therefore use the protected title of 'midwife'. Only the following people may attend a woman in childbirth:*

- *A midwife.*
- *A registered medical practitioner.*
- *A student undergoing training with a view to becoming a midwife or a medical practitioner, as part of an approved course of practical instruction. The exception to this is in a case of 'sudden or urgent necessity'."*

In the Nursing and Midwifery Council (Midwives) Rules Order of Council 2012 (SI 2012 No. 3025), the following definitions are listed: 'Attendance upon' – providing care or advice to a woman or care to a baby whether or not the midwife providing the care or advice is physically present; 'baby' includes an unborn baby during the antenatal and intranatal periods; 'childbirth' includes the antenatal, intranatal and postnatal periods.

8 WHAT ABOUT 'CONCEALING' A PREGNANCY?

Many women worry about being reported to social services for 'concealing a pregnancy'. This concern arises for women if they decide not to engage in medical support while pregnant. This definition appears to be different from Trust to Trust. For example, a review article from Bath Child Health Department by Finlay F, Marcer H and Baverstock A defines concealment of pregnancy as "*one in which a woman knows that she is pregnant but does not tell anyone, or those who are told collude and conceal the fact from health professionals.*"
Whereas an article from Sussex Child protection and safeguarding procedures includes the following in their definition: "*Concealment may be an active act or a form of denial where support of appropriate carers and health professionals is not sought.*"
These definitions are in place to raise safeguarding alerts. This is understandably confusing considering 'concealing' a pregnancy is not an offence. It is an offence

however to conceal a birth under the Offences Against The Person Act 1861. The act states:

> *"If any Woman shall be delivered of a Child, every Person who shall, by any secret Disposition of the dead Body of the said Child, whether such Child died before, at, or after its Birth, endeavour to conceal the Birth thereof, shall be guilty of a Misdemeanour, and being convicted thereof shall be liable, at the Discretion of the Court, to be imprisoned for any Term not exceeding Two Years, with or without Hard Labour: Provided that if any Person tried for the Murder of any Child shall be acquitted thereof, it shall be lawful for the Jury by whose Verdict such Person shall be acquitted to find, in case it shall so appear in Evidence, that the Child had recently been born, and that such Person did, by some secret Disposition of the dead Body of such Child, endeavour to conceal the Birth thereof, and thereupon the Court may pass such Sentence as if such Person had been convicted upon an Indictment for the Concealment of the Birth."*

So should a healthcare professional refer to social services for 'concealment' of a pregnancy? AIMS state the following;

In the UK it is legal for a woman to freebirth her baby and to decline some or all antenatal care. A woman cannot be forced to have anyone present at the birth, nor can she be forced to undergo medical interventions. A woman does not have to justify her decision, nor base it on a particular reason. In the relevant case law for this, Butler-Schloss stated that a woman may refuse medical intervention – which would include antenatal and perinatal care - 'for religious reasons, other reasons, for rational or irrational reasons or for no reason at all.' (See: MB [1997] 8 Med. L.R. *217MB [1997] 8 Med.* L.R. *217 at paragraph 30).*

The only exception to this is when a woman lacks capacity as described by the Mental Capacity Act 2005. However, the Act is very clear in that:

- *every person over 16 is presumed to have capacity unless proven otherwise, and*
- *that a lack of capacity is not proven just because a health carer disagrees with a person's decision or deems it 'unwise.'*

An unassisted pregnancy is an active, legitimate and legal decision to not pursue antenatal care, and it should be respected as such.

This is different from a concealed pregnancy where a woman, frequently vulnerable and experiencing a crisis pregnancy, is concealing her pregnancy from everyone – including friends, family, colleagues etc. In some cases, a woman may be in denial that she is indeed pregnant, or she may be totally unaware of the pregnancy.

As there is ambiguity with the official definition of 'concealing' a pregnancy, this could potentially work in your favour if you are being accused of this. I would suggest you find out how your local trust defines 'concealment'. If you have not concealed your pregnancy from family and friends, or potentially alternative health care providers. You have merely decided not to engage in medical care, which is perfectly legal as it is an OPTIONAL service.

9 POLICY & PROCEDURE FOR SAFEGUARDING FOR HEALTHCARE PROFESSIONALS

If Social Services have been contacted, your healthcare providers might be concerned about the wellbeing of your baby, not just because you have chosen to have an unassisted birth (although this does happen). So what do you do if this has escalated?

Firstly, it is important to make sure the referral has been done correctly. Remember procedure is everything, if a professional has not followed the correct steps, that could be reason enough to dismiss any potential court proceedings.

'Concerns' tend to arise if any of the following 'red flags' are identified during pregnancy. They do not automatically require a referral to Social Services, but they will likely require further discussion between your healthcare provider and their line manager. Consider if your way of living could be perceived as a red flag? For example:

- Mother is unable or unwilling to name the father of her baby
- Domestic abuse or behaviours that suggest there may be a threat to the unborn baby
- Perception that either parent will not be able to care for the baby to an 'acceptable' standard - this may include severe learning difficulties, previous neglect, or living conditions. I would like to point out that acceptable living conditions are subjective to the perceiver. For example, Van life has become very popular, if you live in a van be aware that this may be deemed as unsafe. They may want to see that you have a stable base with running water and heating.
- Mental health problems or drug abuse

10 HOSPITAL CHILD PROTECTION POLICY

Rules within this Policy state that Healthcare Professionals MUST discuss with Parents-to-be, if they are worried about the safety of the baby after birth, unless doing so may put a woman or baby's wellbeing at risk. Healthcare workers should obtain consent before making a referral.
Your trust may vary with specific details, but the following is a typical pathway for professionals assessing and responding to 'concerns' of an unborn baby. If anyof the former mentioned flags are raised, these are the likely steps your healthcare provider will take:

If possible they will want to see the mother alone but cannot actively exclude the father. They will ask about domestic abuse or drug use. Once the pre-birth assessment is complete, there are 3 possible outcomes:

1. Single Agency to support and monitor

2. Multi Agency intervention to ensure mother and baby are supported to achieve the best outcome

- Parents should be informed and discussion should take place where the health provider voices concerns. Consent is not necessary if they believe the baby is in danger

- An early intervention meeting may be held to determine appropriate support

3. Multi Agency intervention is needed to ensure safety of the baby

- If a baby is considered 'in need' which means their basic needs will not be met, MASH (Multi Agency Safeguarding Hub) will likely be contacted . If a baby is considered 'at risk' immediate intervention will take place ie foster care once the baby is born until further investigations are carried out.

- They will complete a MARF (Multi Agency Referral Form) within 24 hours

- If the family in question already have an appointed Social Worker then the referral will be made to them

- Please note - with a 'concealed' pregnancy healthcare workers will likely be told to follow steps for outcome number 3

You can see an example of a safeguarding pathway here https://www.wolverhamptonsafeguarding.org.uk/images/safeguarding-children/children-documents/WSCB_Interagency_Protocol_for_Unborn_Children_and_Young_Children_May_2016.pdf

If social services believe your child is in immediate danger, they can apply for an EPO (Emergency protection order) under section 44 of the Children Act 1989. Usually you will get a one day notice of the application. If they believe the situation to be severe enough, there may be no notice at all.

11 YOUR RIGHTS IF YOU HAVE BEEN REFERRED TO SOCIAL SERVICES

• You have the right to ask to see the full assessment that has taken place. They may not want to produce this but you have the legal right to view any paperwork with relation to your case under the Data Protection Act 2018. If they refuse to provide you with these notes, you have the right to contact the local Social Care Ombudsman and inform them that social services are refusing to disclose your personal records.

• You have the right to know who made the referral. Ask for the name of the person and their PIN number if they are a member of the NMC (ie a nurse of a midwife)
• You do not have to let a social worker into your home if they visit. You should seek legal advice before engaging with them. You will be entitled to legal aid regardless of your financial position.
• Social Services cannot remove your child without a court order or Police Protection order.

12 HOW TO MAKE A COMPLAINT

How to make a complaint

If you believe Social Services have been unnecessarily involved, the first step is to get a full copy of the assessment and/or copies of your pregnancy notes. Find out who reported you (if the individual was a nurse or midwife, find out their PIN number and name) because you can then report them to the NMC for abuse of authority. For example, if you have been reported for an unassisted birth they cannot refer you for this alone. You should contact the NMC and report that individual while simultaneously writing to the Chief Executive of the hospital and consultant midwife with your complaint.

Contact The Autonomy Hotline

When Push Comes To Shove is proud to work with the Autonomy Hotline. This is an amazing organisation of independent specialists in advocacy law, ethics, family life, human rights and medical treatment. They offer outstanding support to those who need it.

0333 772 1227
https://theautonomyhotline.org

13 FINAL THOUGHTS BY BEVERLEY BEECH

Reported or threatened with being reported to Social Services –

Here's what to do.

It is common for women to be threatened with a report to Social Services in order to make them comply with the staff 's requirements: declining treatment either for yourself or your baby is probably the most common.

A threatened report that is not carried through

It is not uncommon for staff to state that if you do not agree with their recommendation then they will have to report you to Social Services. The most common threats relate to: refusing a Vitamin K injection, declining an ultrasound examination, insisting on a home birth. Many women agree as a result of this pressure thereby invalidating the principles of informed consent and against the Code of Practice of their professional bodies. If this has happened to you, you have every right to send a letter or email to the Chief

Executive at the Trust with copies to the Director/Head of Midwifery.

Dear Sir/Madam On the (insert date) I was told by (insert name) that if I did not agree to(insert an explanation of what was threatened) s/he would have to report me to Social Services. Needless to say, this alarmed me considerably and I felt forced to comply (or I refused to comply).
As you are undoubtedly aware, this coercion is unprofessional and contrary to the midwife's/ health visitor's/doctor's Code of Conduct and invalidates and is contrary to the principles of informed consent

I am considering reporting the midwife/health visitor/doctor to their professional body but I would appreciate your comments before I do so.

Note: If you do not have the email address of the Chief Executive you can telephone the hospital and ask to speak to the Chief Executive's secretary and ask her/him for the Chief Executive's email details. A report to Social Services

It is not uncommon for the staff to make an unjustified allegation to Social Services. In which case, it is absolutely necessary to obtain copies of the documentation.

1. Establish who made (or was alleged to have made) the report to Social Services, by writing to the Chief Executive asking for a copy of the telephone record/email/letter that was sent to Social Services about (insert brief details).
2. Write to Social Services stating that you understand that a referral was made to them and asking for a copy of the telephone record/email/letter that prompted their visit.
3. You are entitled to this information under the Freedom of Information Act.

Once you have these details you are in a position to decide what further action to take. The options are: A formal complaint to the Chief Executive at the Trust, a formal complaint to the Nursing and Midwifery Council, the General Medical Council. (Health visitors are registered with the Nursing and Midwifery Council). You may wish to delay this action until your involvement with Social Services is over.

If you would like to discuss this issue feel free to contact Beverley Beech at: beverley.lawrencebeech@gmail.com for further information and advice.

I highly recommend you join us on Telegram if you haven't already.

https://t.me/awakenedbirth

We have the most wonderful community of like minded parents and birth professionals. We are always here to talk if you need support. Please feel free to contact us if you need support throughout your pregnancy and birth journey. We are an alternative maternity service and provide women centred care. We will NEVER tell you what to do or give medical advice, only provide you with evidence based information so you can take control and make informed decisions. We have natural birth practitioners in 6 different countries and even an access fund for low income families.

We provide digital courses from human rights in birth to birth preparation masterclasses! These can be completed at your leisure so you don't have to worry about booking classes with a busy schedule.

If you want to train to be a birth practitioner yourself, we run regular certified courses!

Visit our website now and join the birth revolution! https://www.whenpushcomestoshove.co.uk/

14 REFERENCES

https://blogs.bmj.com/medical-ethics / 2022/01/17/getting-done-for concealment- of-pregnancy-does-a woman-have-a-duty-to-inform healthcare-staff-of-her-preg nancy status/

https:// rotherhamscb.proceduresonline.com / pdfs/app_3_fc_conceal_preg.pdf
https:// rotherhamscb.proceduresonline.com / chapters/p_sg_babies.html

https://cpdonline.co.uk/knowledge base/safeguarding/legislation safeguarding-c hildren/

https://www.nmc.org.uk/globalassets / sitedocuments/nmc-publications/ safeguard ing-policy.pdf

https:// sussexchildprotection.procedures.org . uk/tkyplq

https://www.bathnes.gov.uk/sites/default/files/sitedocuments/Children-and-Young-People/ChildProtection/learning_from_concealed_pregnancy_ final.pdf

https://www.aims.org.uk/information/item/freebirth

https://www.wolverhamptonsafeguarding.org. uk/images/safeguarding-children/children-documents/WSCB_Inter agency_Protocol_for_Unborn_Childre n_and_Young_Children_May_2016.pdf

ABOUT THE AUTHOR

Nickita Starck is founder of When Push Comes To Shove - the fastest growing alternative maternity structure in the world. WPCTS is an EBE award nominated organisation dedicated to empowering women while working closely with The World Council For Health.

Nickita founded the organisation in 2020 when independent midwives in the UK lost their insurance to practice. This was the last hope for women to have autonomy over their birth.

As well as an experienced Natural Birth Practitioner of 13 years, Nickita is also a singer/songwriter and released the song 'Breathe Again' to spread awareness of informed consent in childbirth and her organisation.

Since establishing the organisation Nickita has developed a worldwide network of natural birth practitioners who facilitate non clinical birth.

The message of the movement is simple. Informed consent. Women should give birth in the setting of their choice after making an informed decision. Never to be coerced one way or the other.

Nickita teaches birth physiology to doctors, midwives, doulas and parents-to-be. WPCTS even has an access fund for low income families. No family should be denied care. We rely heavily on generous donations.

Nickita was recently invited to speak at the Better Way Conference in Bath along with some incredible speakers of the truth movement.

To date, Nickita has trained 75 doulas, midwives and doctors and her birth keeper directory spans 6 countries with over 100 practitioners.

Peace on earth will start at birth, if women take control of their birth and are supported in their choices, we will be able to create a better world.

Printed in Great Britain
by Amazon

87776685R00031